Yes, I Can.

I Can Do Anything!

Yes, I Can.

I Can Do Anything!

By Tobi Pavlas

Illustrations by Allyson Taylor

ISBN: 978-1-7330393-9-0

ISBN: 1-7330393-9-2

Library of Congress Control Number: 2019907673

Illustrations by: Allyson Taylor

Sacred Life Publishers™

SacredLife.com
Printed in the United States of America

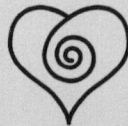

Dedicated to
My Ness

Abel was a typical nine-year-old boy who loved to play. The only thing different about Abel was that he used a wheelchair to move around. His wheelchair had slanted wheels, cool racing stickers, and decals.

This particular morning, he was excited about it being the first day of school. He woke up . . .

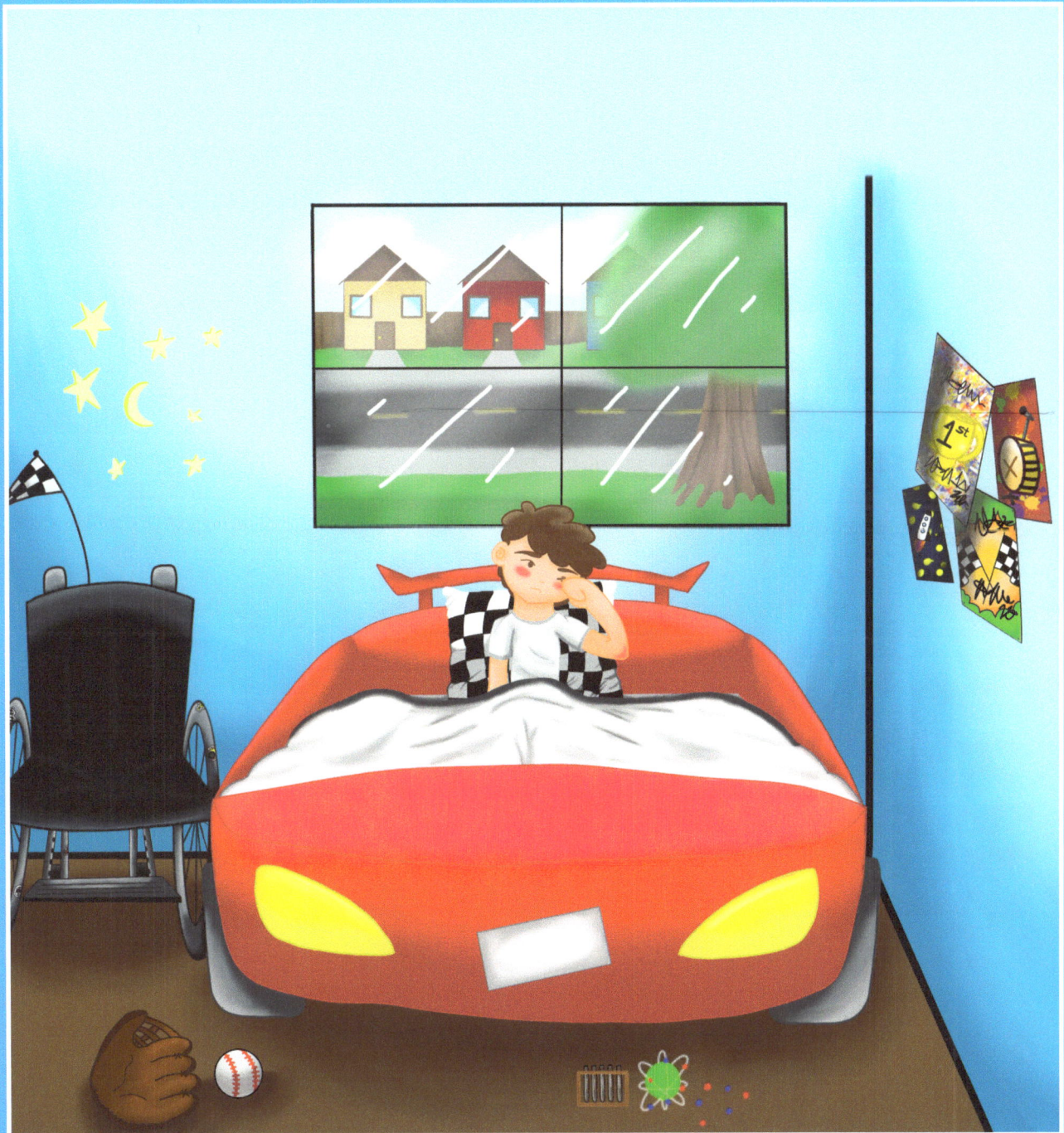

. . . had some breakfast,

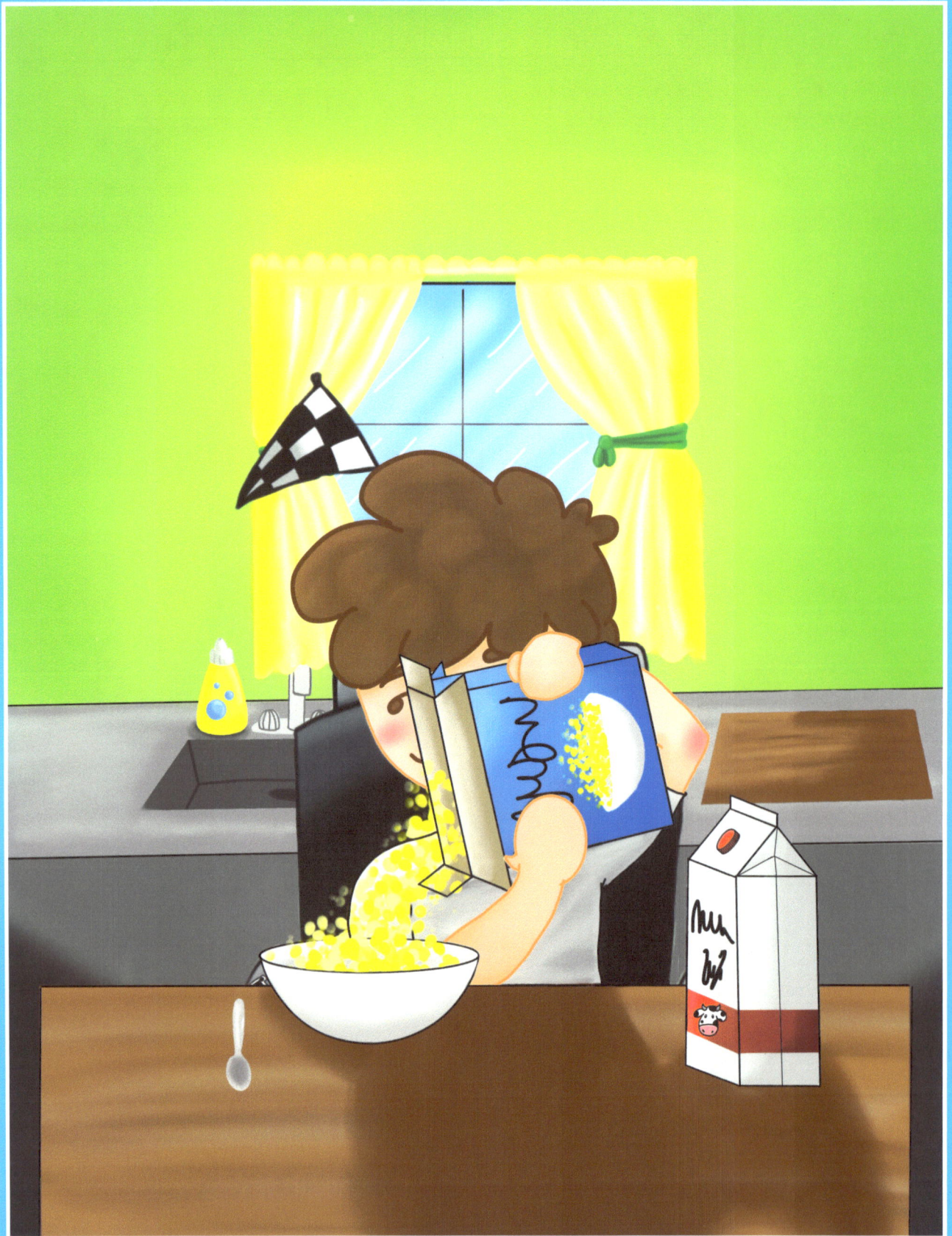

. . . brushed his teeth,

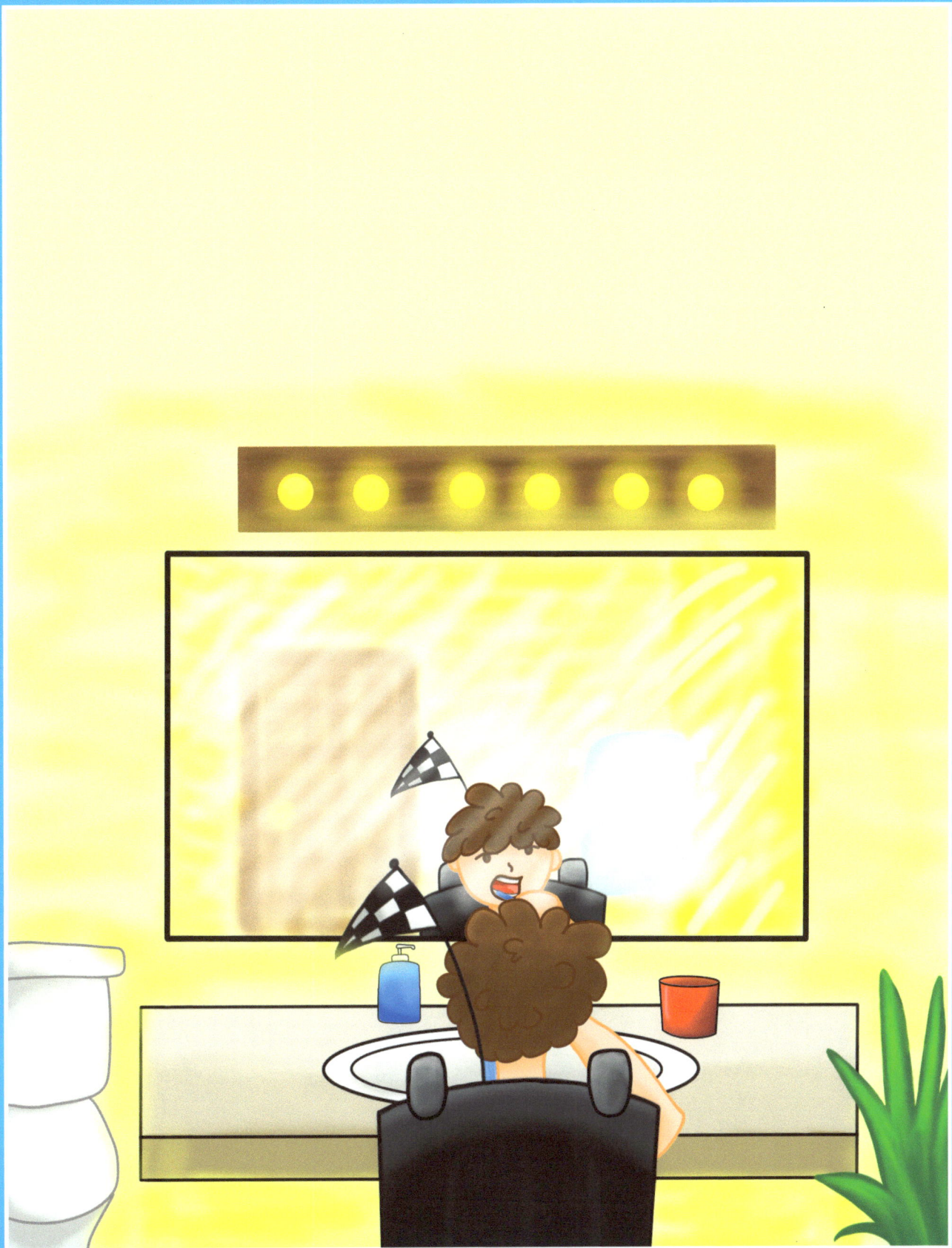

. . . and, got dressed for school.

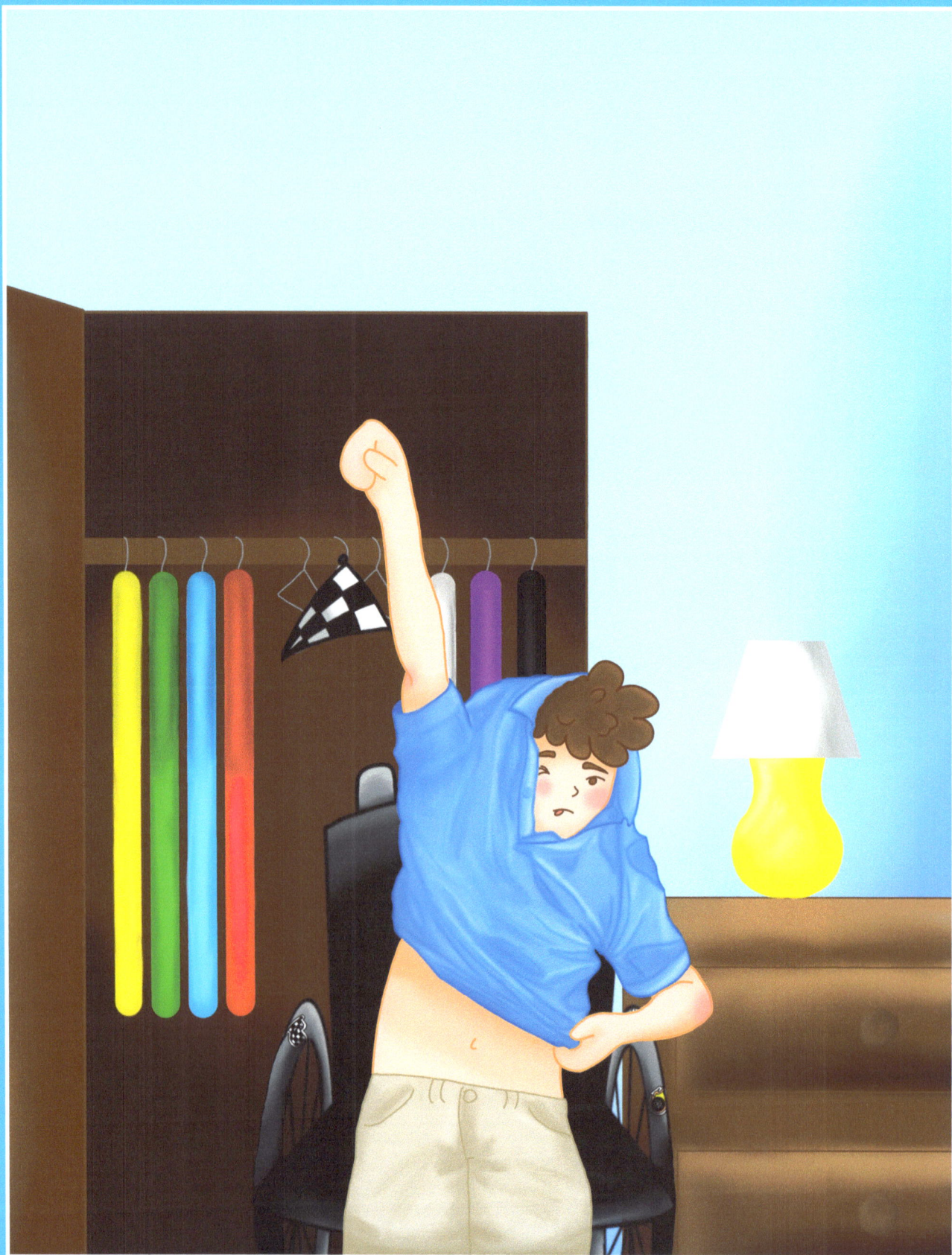

4

Just as she had done since first grade, Abel's neighbor and close friend Sally arrived at his door so they could go to school together. On the way, Abel and Sally passed the baseball field where some boys were playing a game. Abel thought it looked like fun, so he asked if he could play. One of the boys, whose name was Chance, replied, "You can't run the bases!"

Abel looked at Chance, smiled, and replied, *"Yes, I can. I can do anything!"*

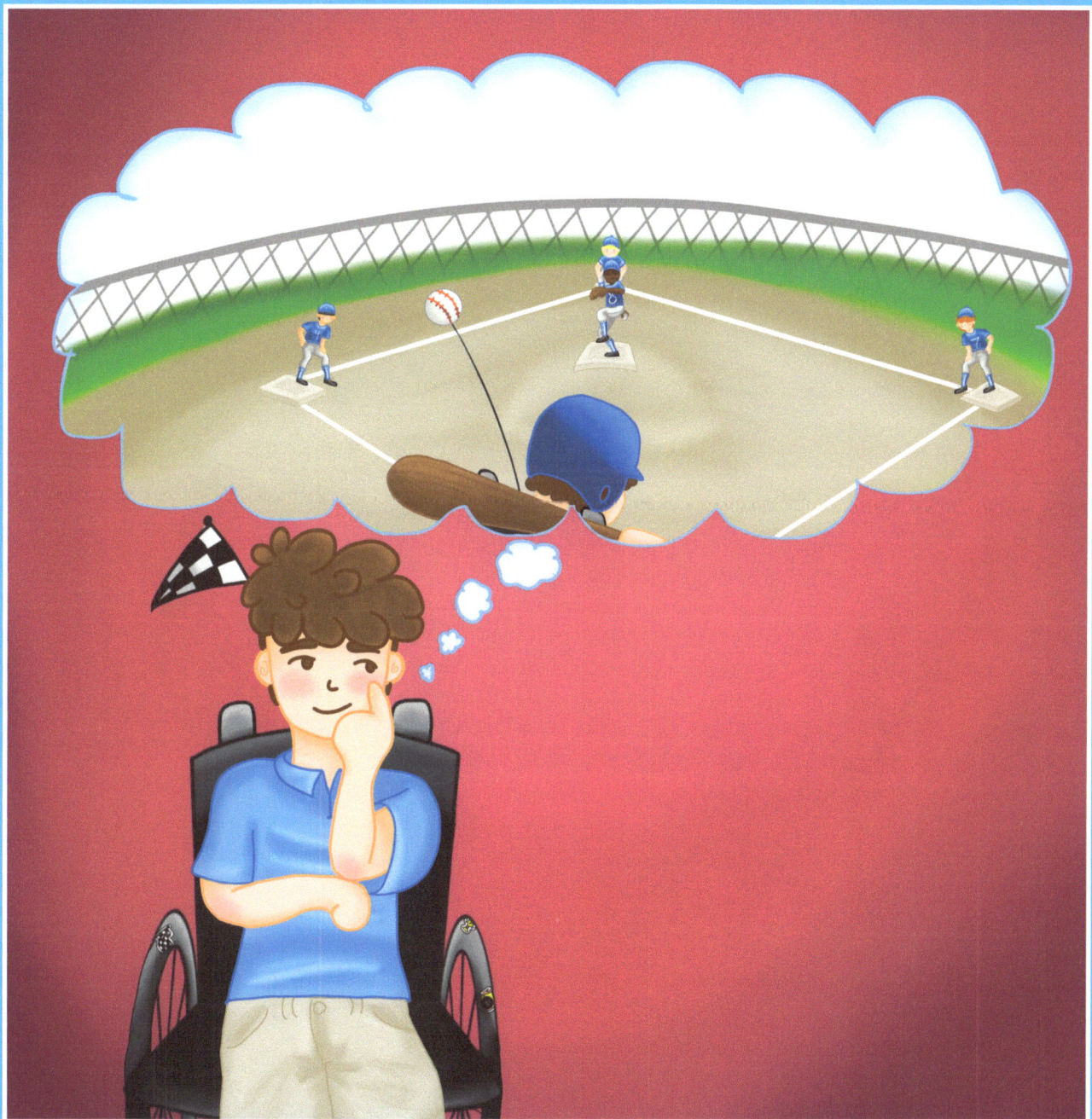

Chance let Abel play and watched as Abel sent the ball flying high. He dropped the bat and sped to first base.

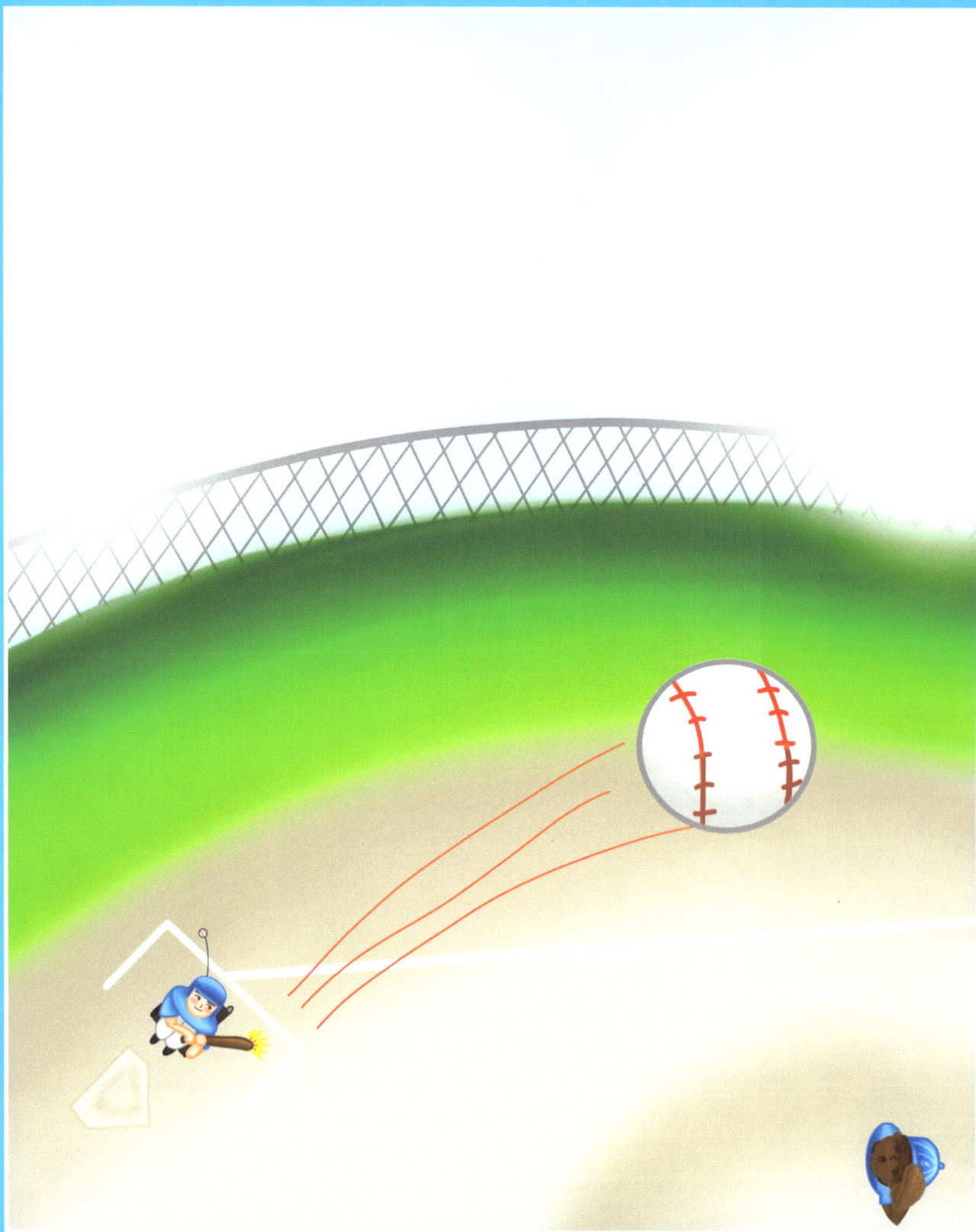

Sally cheered for her friend and then noticed the time. "Abel," she called out, "We shouldn't be late for the first day! We have to go!"

Abel gave Sally a high five as he prepared to leave the field. Chance yelled after them, "Abel, can you play baseball with us next week when we play our first official game?"

"Thanks," Abel replied. "That would be fun!"

Abel and Sally arrived at school on time. Sally was in Mrs. Green's class, and Abel was in Mr. Kent's class, so they said goodbye and that they would see each other at recess.

On the playground during recess, some of the kids were playing Space Station. Abel asked if he could join. Sally stood by the hopscotch court, observing the other kids. Bobby, a fifth-grader, looked at Abel and told him, "You can't be an astronaut!"

Abel replied, *"Yes, I can. I can do anything."*

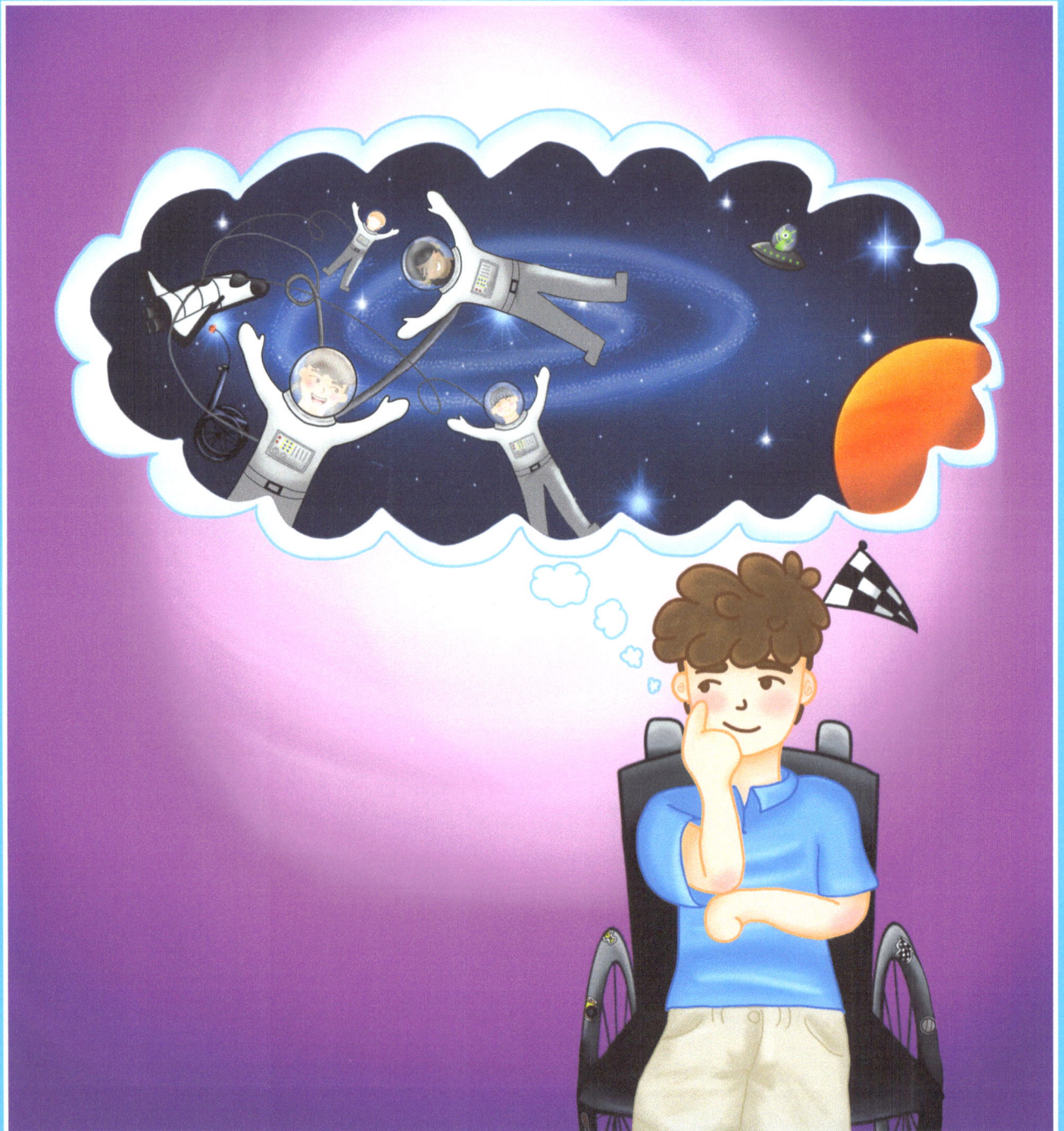

Bobby and his group admired Abel's confidence and invited him to join them. They watched in wonder as Abel used his wheelchair controls to serve as the control panel for the Space Station.

"We need to reposition the satellite," Abel proclaimed, using his most adult voice. "We need to reprogram the coordinates! Command, what are your orders?"

Sally, joined in. "Come in, Commander Abel. The coordinates are fifteen degrees south and two hundred degrees north east."

The boys happily complied with Abel's commands, enjoying their new friend's imagination. Just when the spaceship was about to land, the bell rang. Recess was over.

Before Abel sped off, Bobby asked hopefully, "Abel, can you come finish our space mission tomorrow? It was fun playing with you today!"

Abel smiled. "Sure, see you then!"

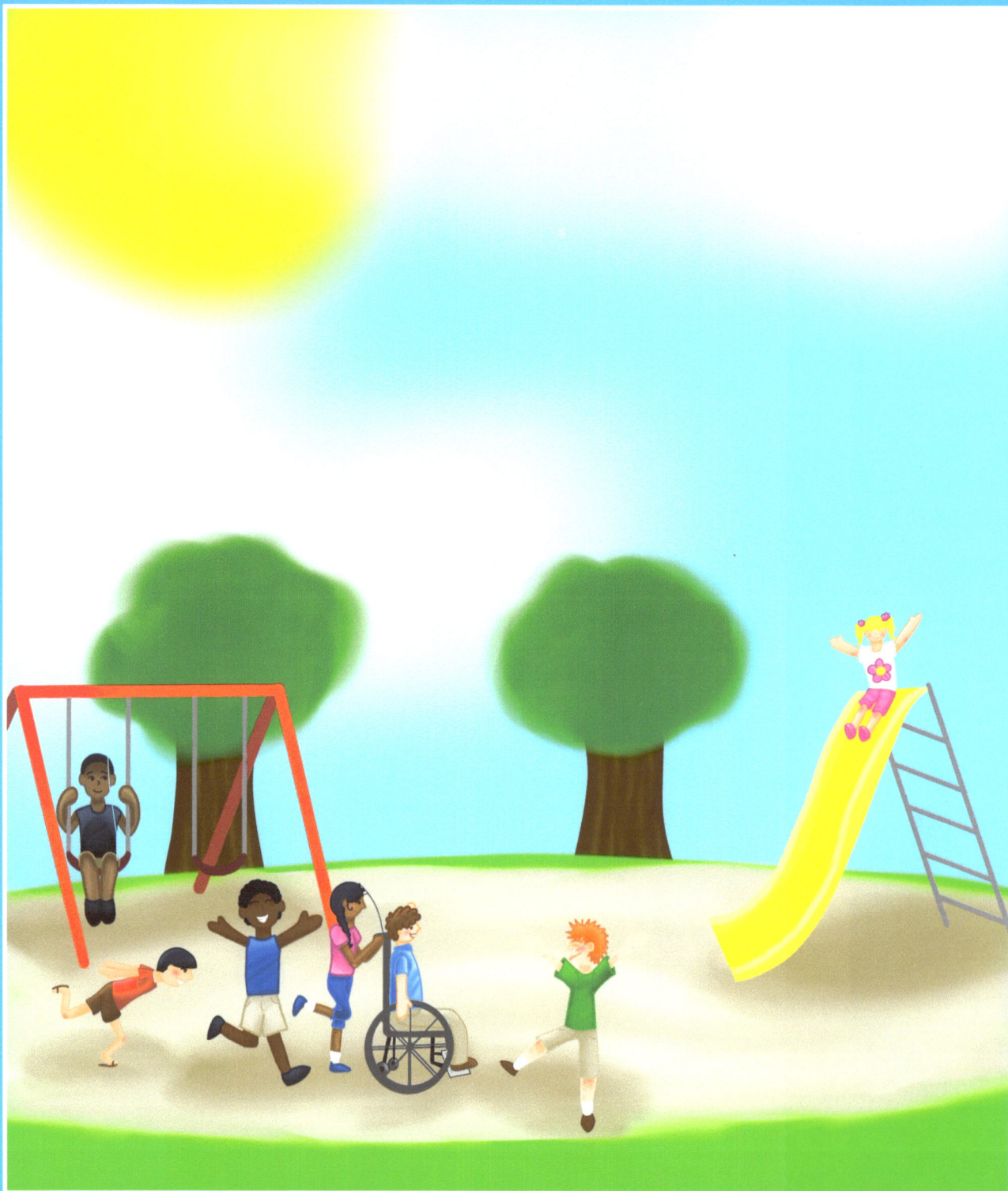

At lunchtime, Abel met Sally in the cafeteria. A song from Abel's favorite rock band was playing through the cafeteria speakers. A few girls from Sally's class were singing and dancing to the music. Abel asked to join them. One of the girls, Chloe, informed him, "You can't be a rockstar!"

Smiling, Abel, replied, "*Yes, I can. I can do anything!*"

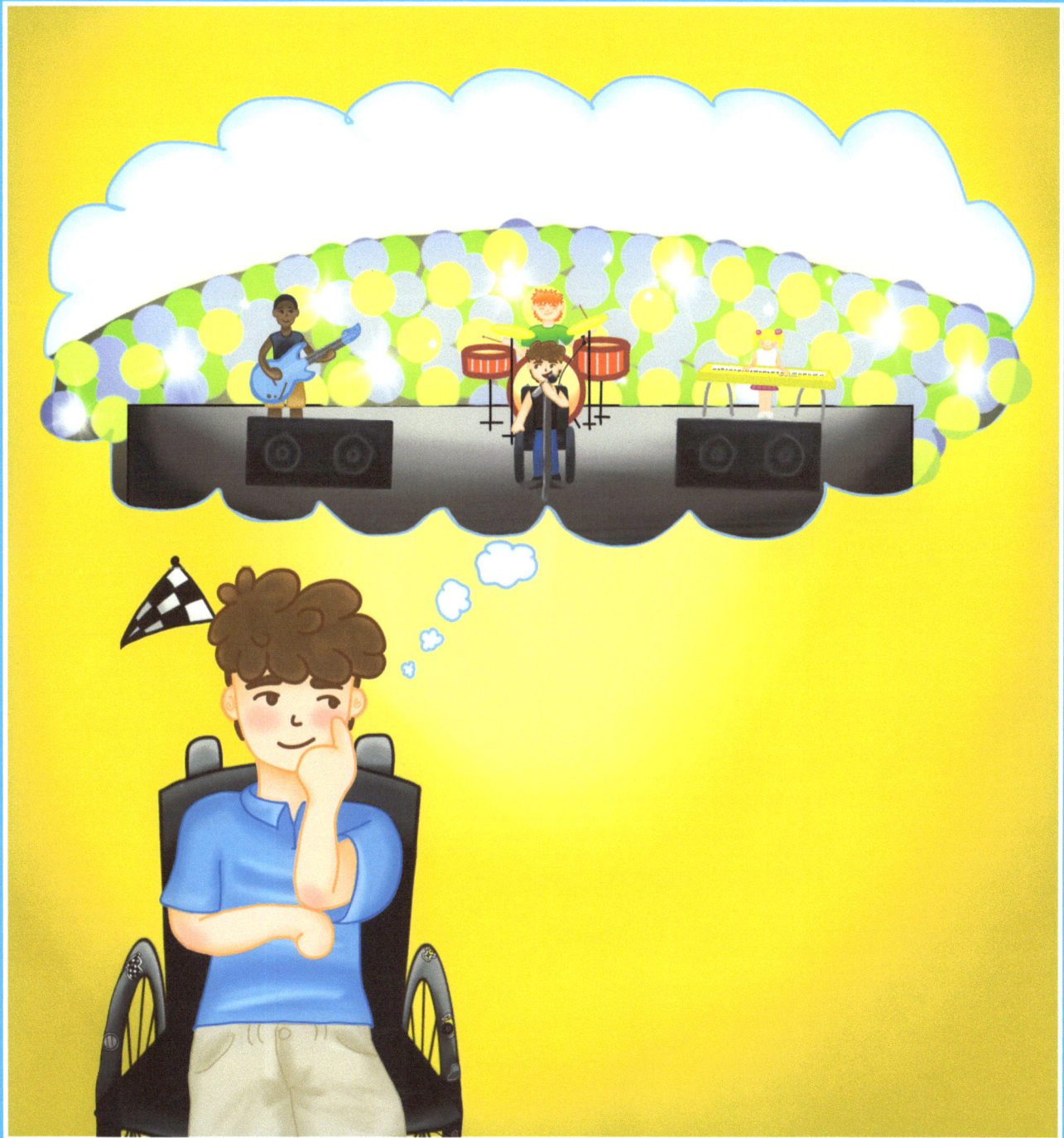

Chloe watched with amazement as a fearless Abel used his milk carton for a microphone! Grabbing Sally's hand, Chloe and the girls started singing and swaying behind him to the music. Together, they all performed the best rock concert, ever!

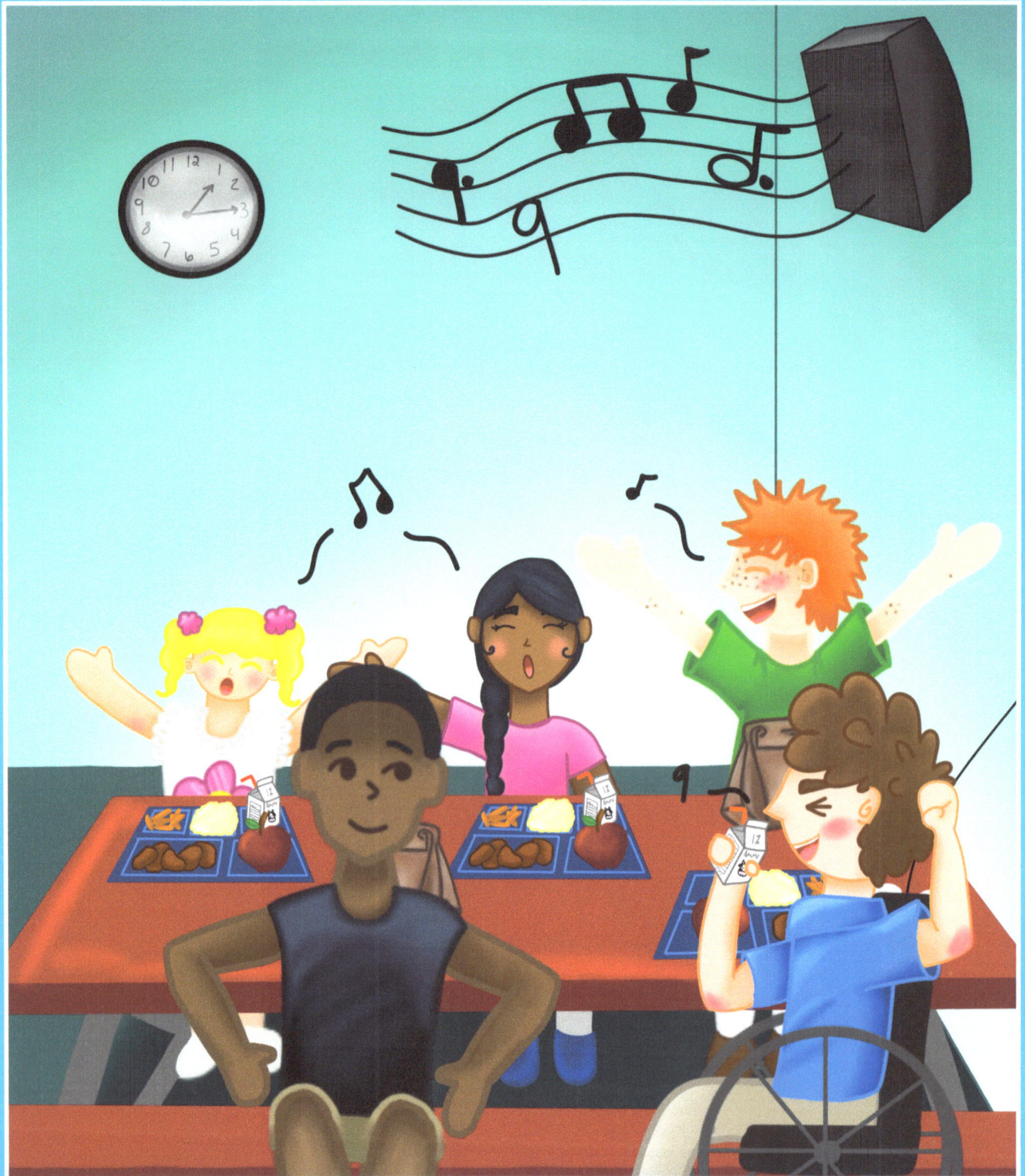

Once the bell rang, the kids started heading back to class. Chloe smiled at her new friend and said, "I could sing with you *any day*, Abel."

Abel grinned at Chloe and bowed in his chair.

At the end of the day, Sally and Abel cruised by the playground as they started the journey home. Abel recognized Oscar and a few other kids from his class playing in the sandbox.

Abel, called out, "What are you doing? Can I play?" Oscar looked at Abel's wheelchair, "We're playing Science Lab. You can't be a scientist!"

Abel calmly told him, *"Yes, I can. I can do anything."*

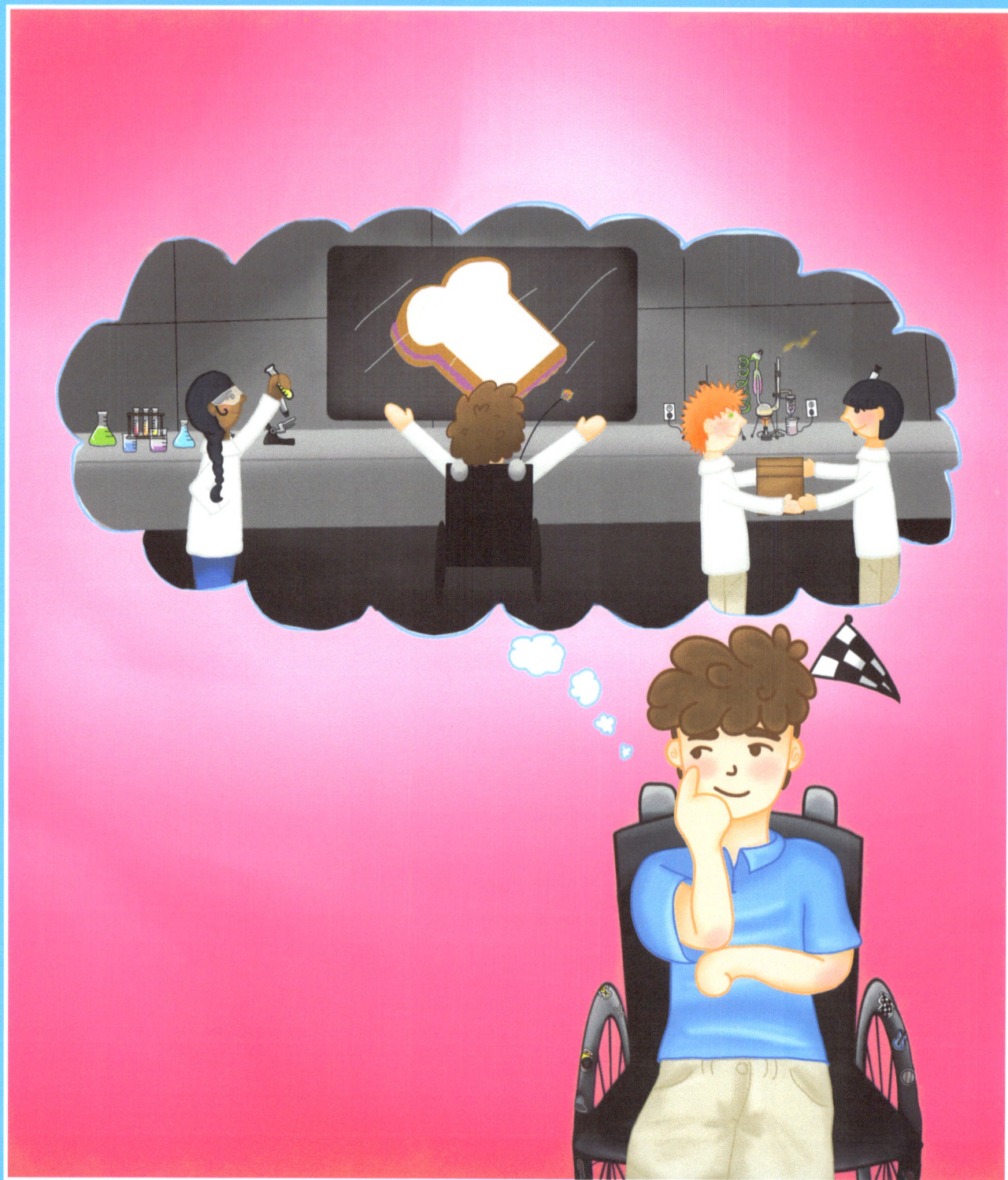

Oscar watched, fascinated, as Abel gathered sand and small rocks into his empty water bottle. Using a clear pencil sharpener as a magnifying glass, Abel pretended to examine the mixture and take notes about chemical reactions. "We must add some blue compound, and then the medicine should be complete and ready for testing," Abel concluded.

Sally joined her friends and took a ruler out of her backpack. She pretended to measure the water bottle full of sand and said, "This should be the correct potion. All we need now are test subjects."

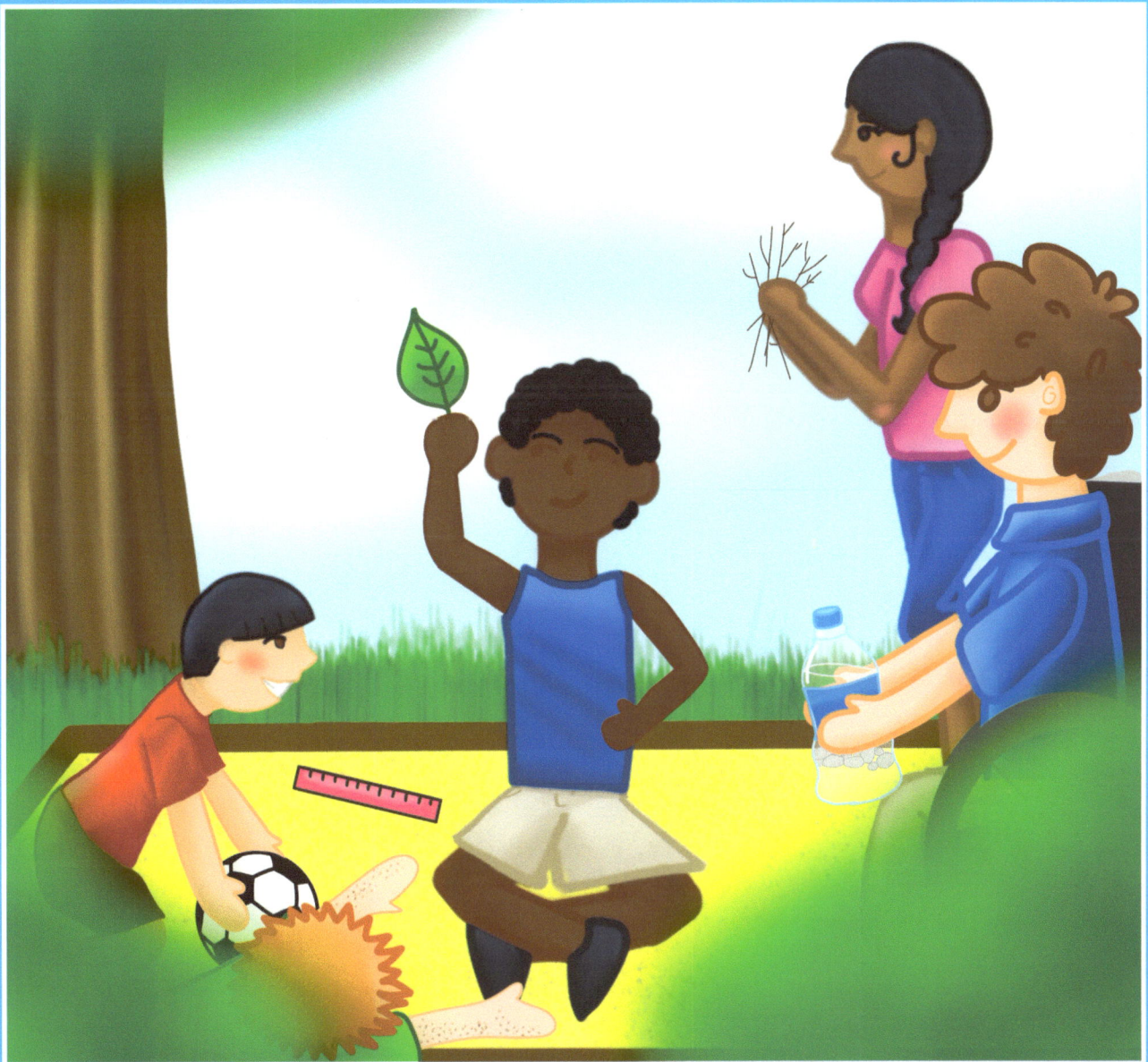

Once the medicine was safe and approved, Abel and Sally had to return home. Oscar patted Abel on the back and said, "Maybe you can play with us tomorrow?"

Abel gave Oscar a knuckle bump. He answered, "Yes, I can," and said goodbye to his new friend.

On the way home Sally told Abel, "I'm glad we had so much fun together."

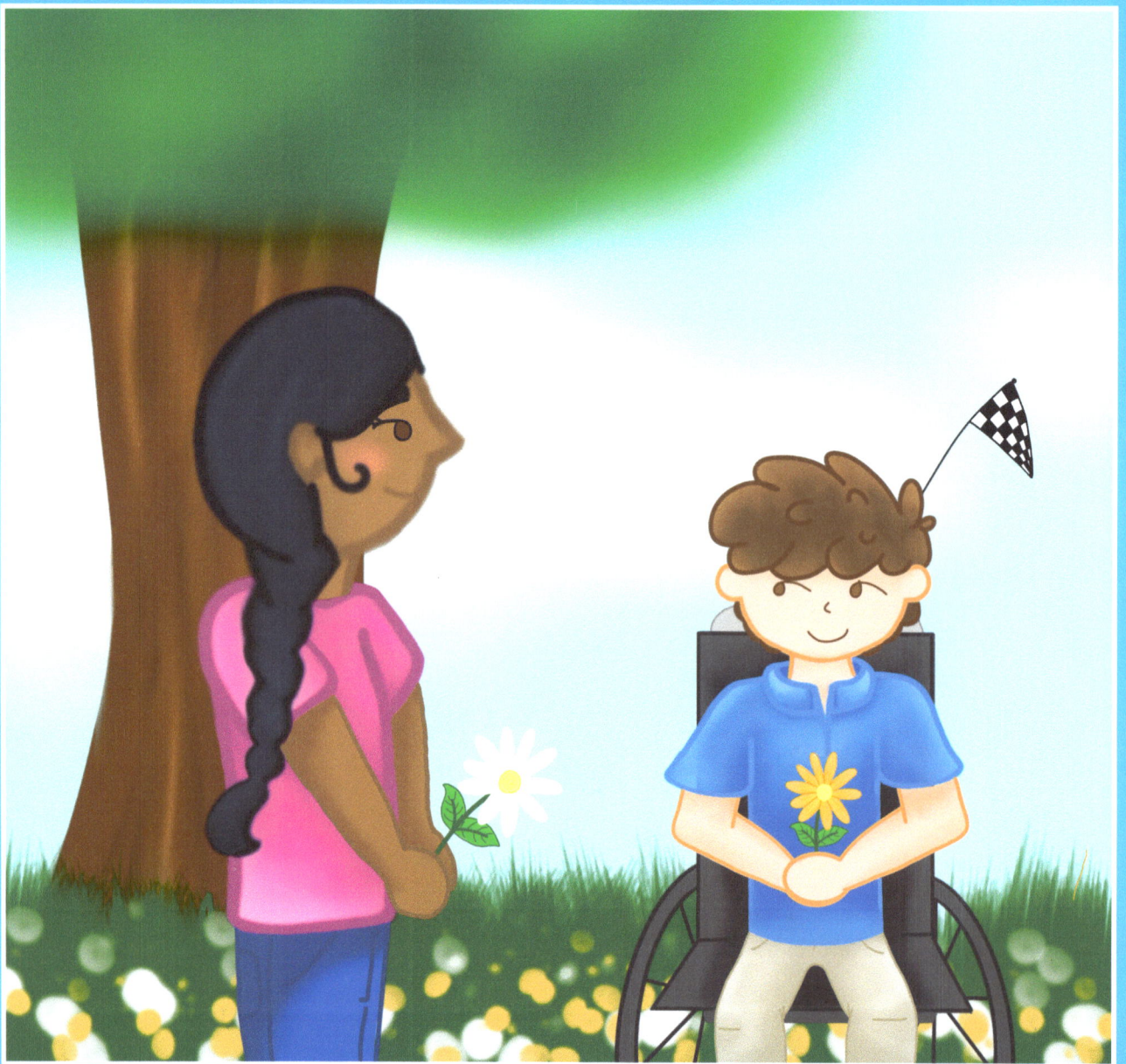

Once they reached Abel's house, Sally told her best friend, "Today was fun! I'll see you in the morning."

Abel watched as she skipped away and called after her excitedly, "Bye, Sally!"

Sally waved goodbye.

Abel wheeled up the ramp to his house and let himself inside. As he set down his backpack, his mom greeted her son with a smile. "How was your first day?"

Abel grabbed an apple out of the fruit bowl. "It was great, Mom. I made some new friends, and we played together. I was a baseball player, an astronaut, a rockstar, and a scientist!"

His mom was not surprised. Proud of Abel, she hugged him. "How wonderful! I'll call you when dinner's ready."

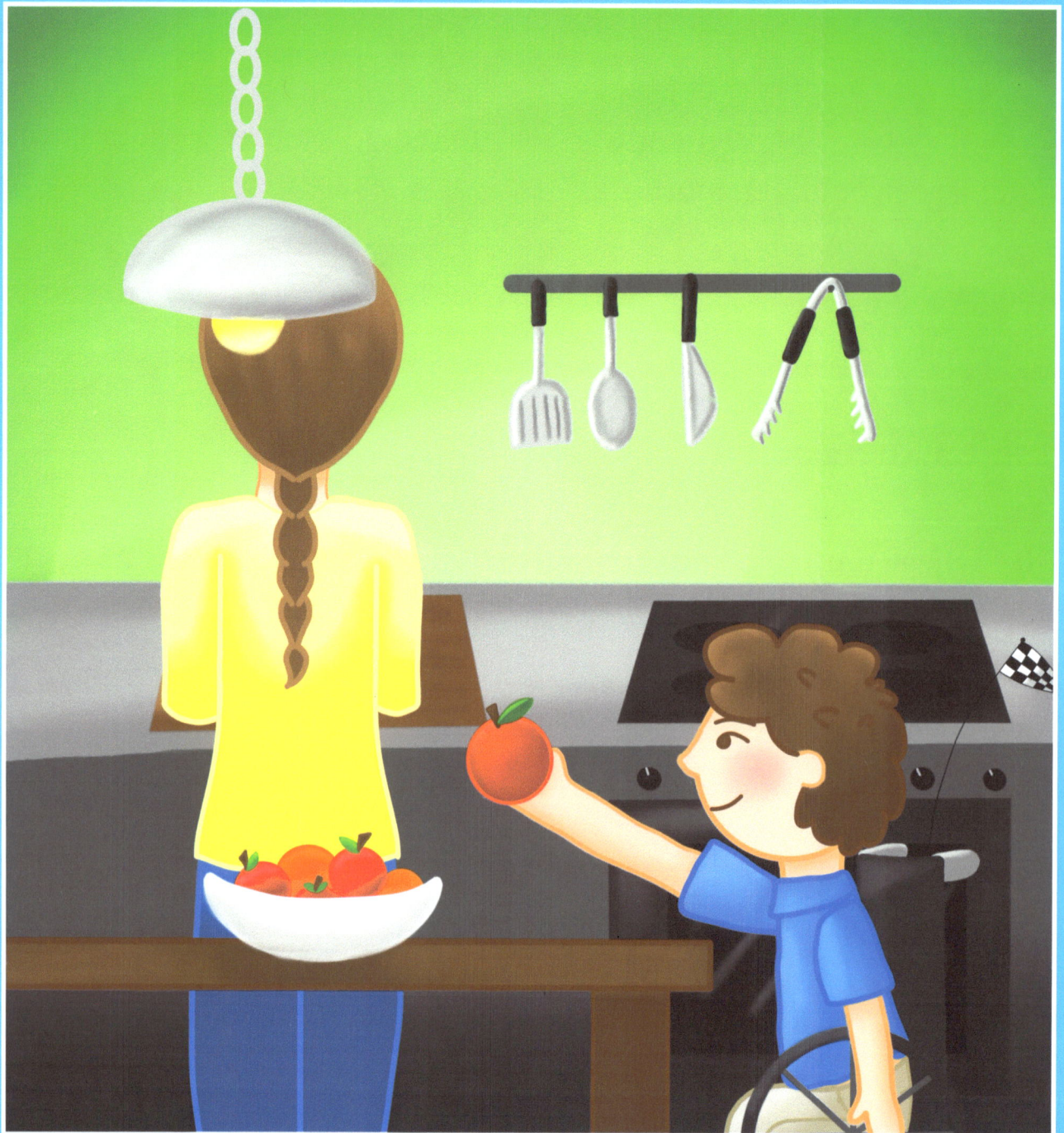

After doing his homework,

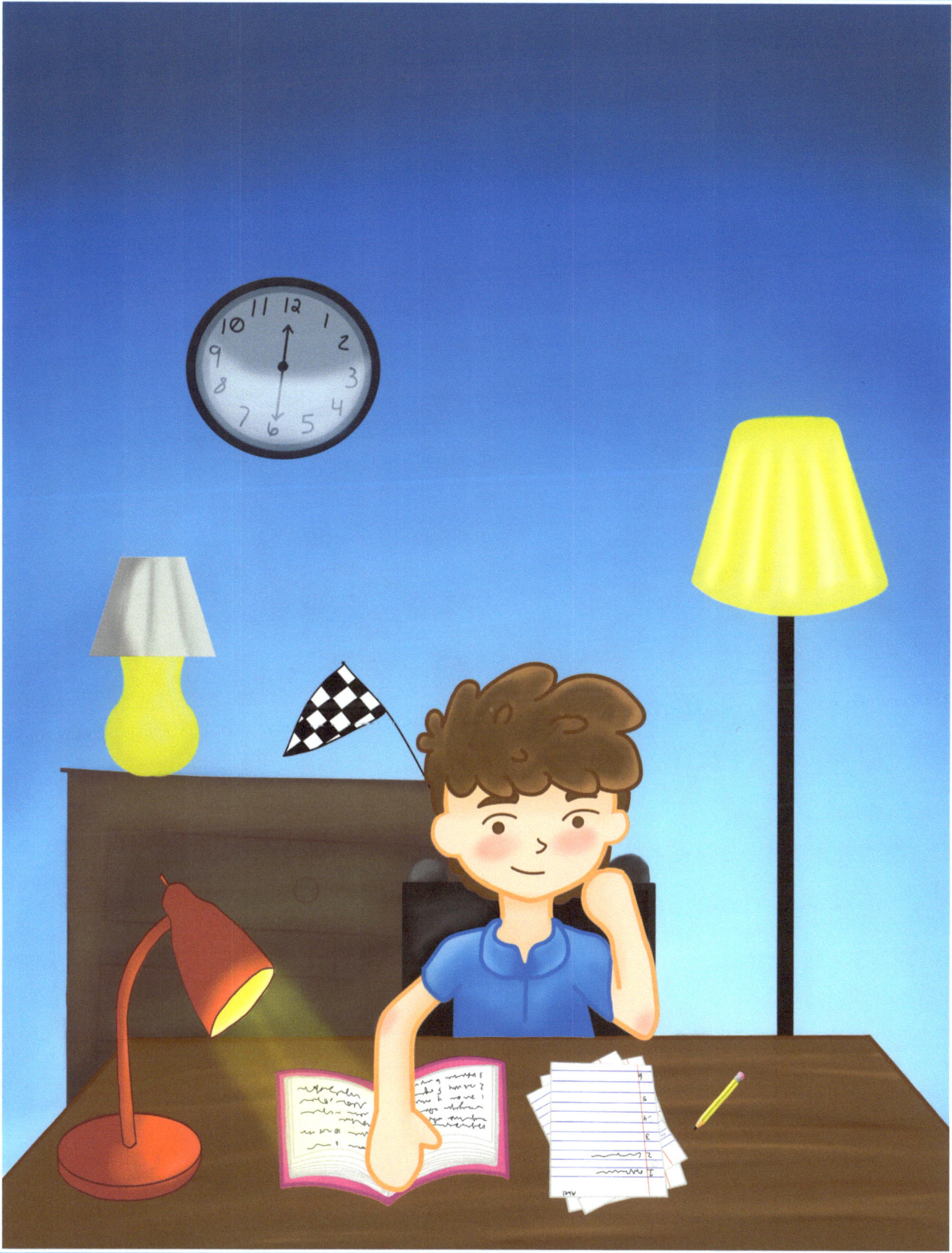

. . . eating dinner,

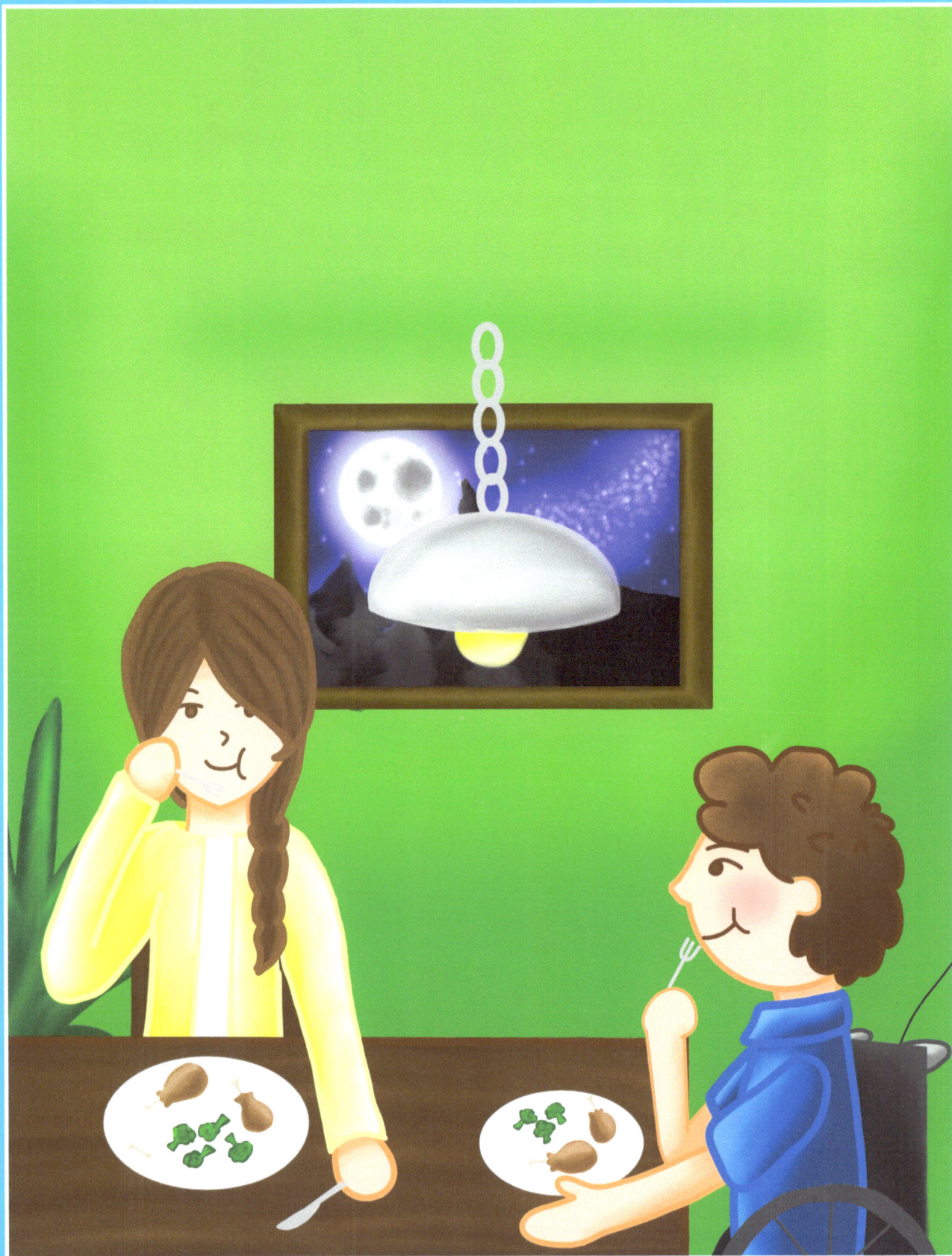

. . . and some chores,

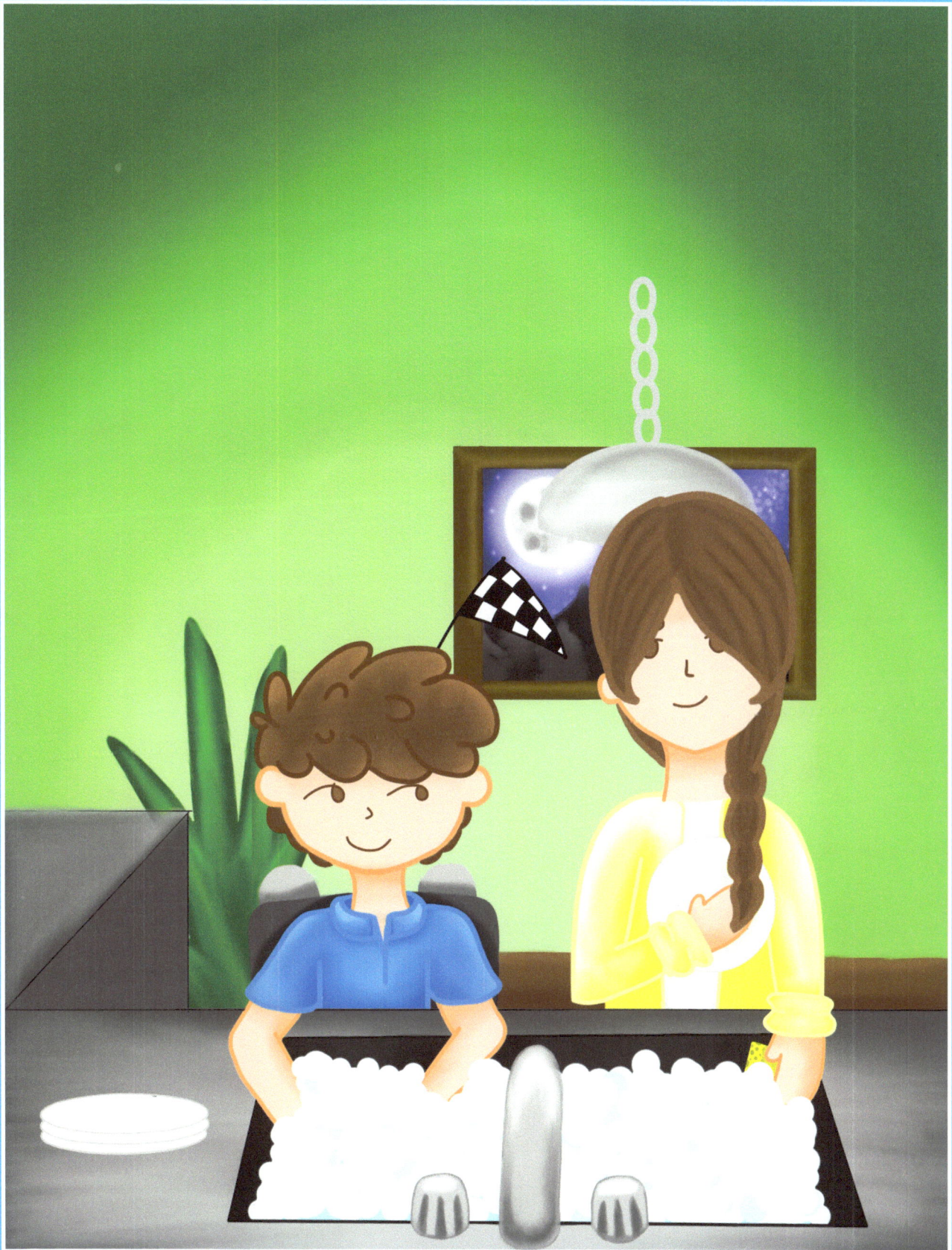

. . . it was time for bed. Abel was tired after an exciting first day of school. After all, being a baseball player, an astronaut, a rockstar, and a scientist—all in one day—wasn't easy! He couldn't wait to go back to school and play with all of the new friends he had made.

When his mother came in to say good night, she kissed him on his sleepy head.

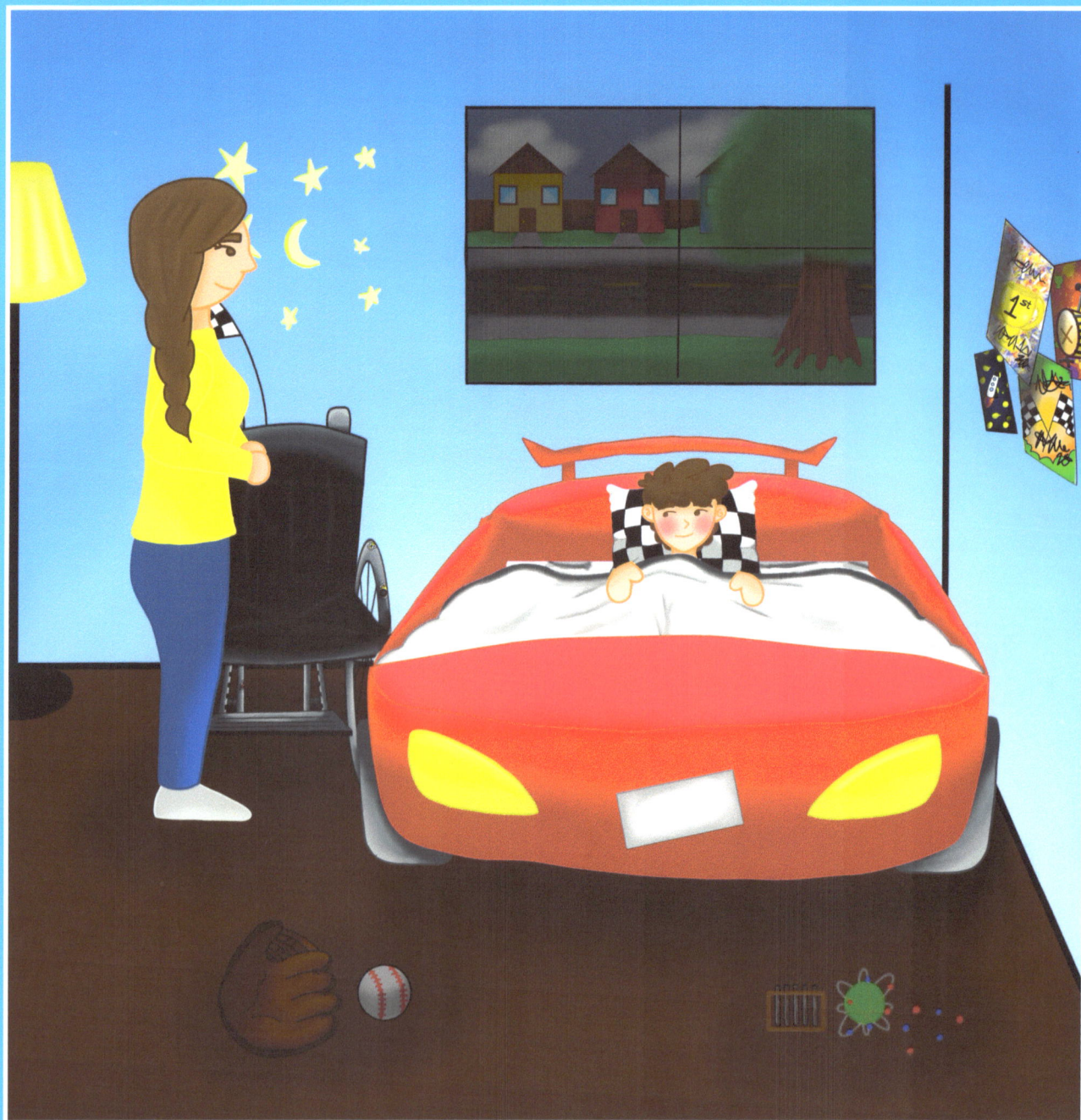

Abel yawned and closed his eyes as she tucked him into bed.

Before leaving his room, she whispered in his ear, "Remember, Abel, you can do anything."

Abel's mom turned off his light and closed his door, smiling at the stickers that decorated it. Grateful for the blessing who was her son, she whispered to herself, "And, I know you will."

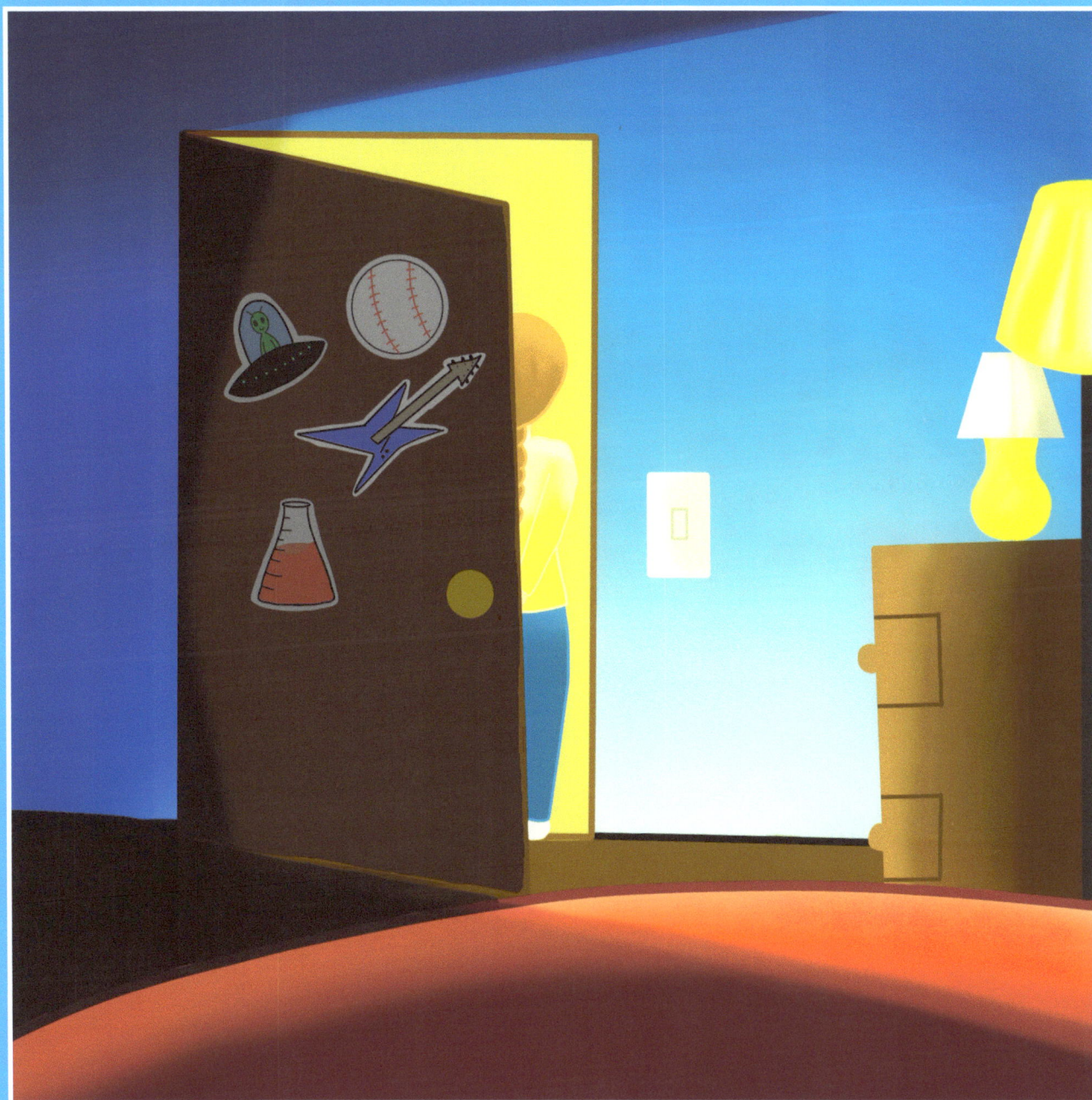

Acknowledgments

Oh Cappy, my Cappy, I thank you for your advice and encouragement.

To the Pilates Guru, thanks for nudging me when I needed it.

To my womb mate, I cherish you.

www.ingramcontent.com/pod-product-compliance
Lightning Source LLC
Chambersburg PA
CBHW061355090426

42739CB00002B/31